MIGRAINE RELIEF PLAN AND COOKBOOK

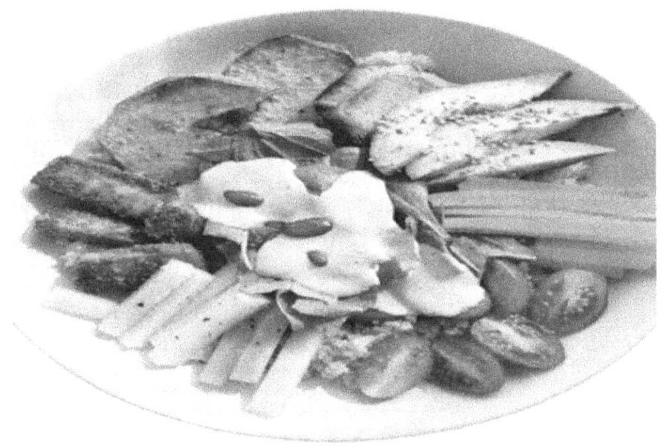

A simple and effective way on how to prevent and reduce pain, inflammation and stress with Anti-inflammatory recipes and strategies to stop migraines.

KATHLEEN G MARION

TABLE OF CONTENT

INTRODUCTION

Jay, a vibrant architect with a passion for life, was plagued by an unwelcome shadow: chronic migraines. Throbbing temples, nausea, and an aversion to light transformed simple days into struggles. He tried everything – prescription meds, blackout curtains, even acupuncture. While some offered fleeting relief, none delivered lasting freedom. Frustration gnawed at him, whispering that life under a migraine cloud was his fate.

One dreary afternoon, amidst towering stacks of blueprints and a pounding headache, Jay stumbled upon a glimmer of hope - **your migraine relief plan and cookbook**. Skeptical but desperate, he dove into the pages. What unfolded wasn't just a collection of recipes, but a roadmap to a life reclaimed.

He learned about the science behind migraines, discovering how specific foods could be triggers, lurking in his seemingly healthy meals. The book wasn't a restrictive tyrant, but a guide, offering delicious alternatives. He swapped his morning bagel, often a culprit, for a protein-packed omelet bursting with spinach and peppers. Lunch became a symphony of colorful salads, drizzled with flavorful vinaigrettes, instead of his usual greasy sandwiches. Dinner transformed into a culinary adventure, exploring dishes rich in fruits, vegetables, and lean proteins.

Initially, adjustments were bumpy. He craved his old favorites, the familiar comfort of routine. But with each migraine-free day, his resolve grew. He discovered hidden gems – the tangy sweetness of roasted sweet potatoes, the creamy comfort of cashew-based sauces. His taste buds danced, his body thrived.

The change wasn't just physical. The mental fog lifted, replaced by a clarity he hadn't known in years. He could work longer, laugh more deeply, engage with life with an unburdened heart. He became a culinary crusader, sharing his newfound knowledge with friends and family, witnessing their own transformations. He even started a blog, chronicling his journey and inspiring others.

One sun-drenched afternoon, while sketching a new design, Jay realized he hadn't had a migraine in months. He looked at the vibrant cookbook, no longer a beacon of hope, but a testament to his victory. He had rewritten his story, not just on paper, but on his plate, proving that sometimes, the tastiest recipe is the one for a life free from pain. His story became a beacon, encouraging others to embark on their own culinary crusades against migraines, proving that delicious food and well-being could go hand in hand.

Jay's journey is a testament to the transformative power of your cookbook. It's not just a collection of recipes; it's a key unlocking a world where flavor and well-being dance in perfect harmony. So, pick up your copy, embark on your own culinary adventure, and rewrite your story, one delicious bite at a time.

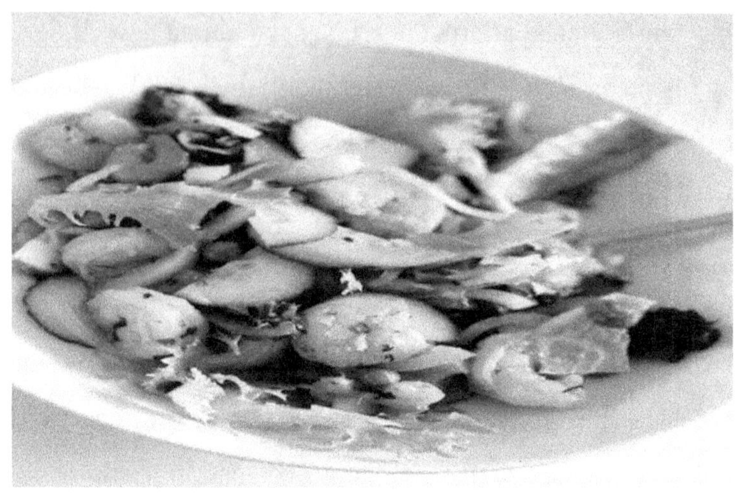

CHAPTER 1

Your Comprehensive Guide to Migraines, Relief, and Delicious Solutions

Imagine a world where throbbing headaches don't hold your hostage, where vibrant colors don't trigger blinding waves of pain, and where every day presents an opportunity to thrive. For millions battling migraines, such a world often feels more like a distant dream. But what if that dream could become reality?

This comprehensive guide, inspired by your **Migraine Relief Plan and Cookbook**, delves into the complex world of migraines, empowering you with knowledge, practical solutions, and delicious pathways to alleviate discomfort and reclaim your life.

Understanding the Foe: Unveiling the Types of Migraines

Migraines aren't just one-size-fits-all headaches. They manifest in various forms, each with its own characteristics:

- **Migraine with Aura:** This type boasts visual disturbances like shimmering lights, blind spots, or tingling sensations before the head pain arrives.
- **Migraine without Aura:** The most common type, featuring intense throbbing pain on one side of the head, often accompanied by nausea, vomiting, and sensitivity to light and sound.
- **Chronic Migraine:** Defined by experiencing 15 or more migraine days per month, lasting for at least 3 months.
- **Hemiplegic Migraine:** A rare yet severe form causing temporary weakness or paralysis on one side of the body.
- **Basilar Migraine:** Affecting the brainstem, it triggers dizziness, vertigo, tinnitus, and potentially slurred speech.

A Labyrinth of Causes: Unveiling the Triggers

While the exact cause of migraines remains a mystery, research unveils a complex interplay of factors:

- **Genetics:** Studies indicate a strong hereditary component, with certain genes increasing susceptibility.
- **Brain Chemicals:** Fluctuations in neurotransmitters like serotonin and glutamate are thought to play a role.
- **Triggers:** Specific external factors can ignite a migraine attack, including stress, hormonal changes, and lack of sleep, certain foods, weather changes, and strong smells.

Identifying the Enemy's Weapons: Recognizing Symptoms

The telltale signs of a migraine vary, but common symptoms include:

- **Intense throbbing pain:** Often on one side of the head, sometimes migrating or changing intensity.
- **Nausea and vomiting:** Feeling queasy and potentially throwing up during an attack.
- **Sensitivity to light and sound:** Bright lights and loud noises can exacerbate the pain.
- **Aura:** The visual disturbances or tingling sensations experienced in migraines with aura.
- **Fatigue:** Feeling drained and exhausted before, during, and after an attack.
- **Mood changes:** Irritability, depression, or anxiety can occur before or during a migraine.

Fortifying Your Defenses: Preventive Measures

While there's no guaranteed cure, proactive steps can significantly reduce the frequency and severity of migraine attacks:

- **Identify and avoid triggers:** Keep a headache diary to track potential triggers and create personalized avoidance strategies.
- **Maintain a regular sleep schedule:** Aim for 7-8 hours of quality sleep each night.
- **Manage stress:** Explore relaxation techniques like yoga, meditation, or deep breathing exercises.
- **Stay hydrated:** Drink plenty of water throughout the day to avoid dehydration, a potential trigger.
- **Eat a healthy diet:** Choose nutrient-rich foods and limit processed foods, sugary drinks, and excessive caffeine.
- **Regular exercise:** Engage in physical activity most days of the week, but avoid strenuous exercise right before bed.
- **Medications:** Preventive medications prescribed by your doctor can help reduce the frequency or intensity of migraines.

The Culinary Crusade: Harnessing Food as Your Ally

Now, let's unlock the secrets of your **Migraine Relief Plan and Cookbook**, where food becomes your secret weapon against migraines. This book goes beyond bland restrictions, offering a delicious and effective approach to migraine management through targeted nutrition:

- **Anti-inflammatory Diet:** Prioritizing fruits, vegetables, whole grains, lean protein, and healthy fats, minimizing inflammatory foods like processed meats, sugary drinks, and refined carbohydrates.
- **Recipes Tailored to Your Needs:** Discover a symphony of dishes catering to diverse dietary preferences, offering delicious alternatives to potential triggers.
- **Meal Plans:** Take the guesswork out of healthy eating with weekly plans designed to support your migraine management journey.
- **Expert Guidance:** Gain insights from medical professionals and chefs, empowering you to navigate dietary choices with confidence.

Remember, you're not alone in this battle. By understanding the types of migraines, their causes and symptoms, and embracing preventive measures, you can build a strong defense. Additionally, your **Migraine Relief Plan and Cookbook** offers a delicious and empowering culinary arsenal to manage your migraines and reclaim your life. Together, knowledge, proactive measures, and the power of food can turn your migraine challenges into stepping stones towards a healthier, happier you.

CHAPTER 2

Navigate the Delicious Labyrinth: Foods to Embrace and Avoid in Your Migraine Relief Plan

Migraines can be debilitating, robbing you of precious moments and impacting your overall well-being. While the exact cause remains elusive, research continues to unveil the intricate dance between food and migraine triggers. Your **Migraine Relief Plan and Cookbook** unlocks the secrets of this dance, offering a practical guide to navigate the food landscape and empower your journey towards optimal health.

Embracing Anti-Inflammatory Allies:

Imagine a vibrant plate bursting with colors, packed with nutrients – your anti-inflammatory haven. These ingredients become your allies in combating migraines, reducing inflammation and supporting overall well-being:

- **Fruits and Vegetables:** Nature's powerhouses, rich in antioxidants and vitamins, like berries, leafy greens, peppers, and citrus fruits.
- **Whole Grains:** Choose brown rice, quinoa, oats, and whole-wheat bread for sustained energy and fiber.
- **Lean Protein:** Opt for skinless chicken, fish, beans, lentils, and tofu for essential nutrients without inflammatory effects.
- **Healthy Fats:** Embrace avocados, nuts, seeds, and olive oil as sources of good fats crucial for brain health.
- **Spices and Herbs:** Explore the anti-inflammatory properties of turmeric, ginger, garlic, and rosemary to add flavor and boost your health.

Farewell to Migraine Triggers:

While every individual's trigger landscape is unique, certain ingredients are known to contribute to migraine attacks. Identifying and minimizing these foods empowers you to take control:

- **Processed Meats:** Hot dogs, sausages, and deli meats often contain nitrates and nitrites, potential migraine triggers.

- **Refined Carbohydrates:** White bread, sugary cereals, and pastries cause blood sugar spikes linked to migraines.
- **Aged Cheeses:** Cheddar, blue cheese, and Parmesan contain tyramine, an amino acid implicated in migraines for some individuals.
- **Monosodium Glutamate (MSG):** This flavor enhancer found in processed foods and Chinese cuisine can trigger migraines in sensitive individuals.
- **Artificial Sweeteners:** Aspartame and sucralose, commonly used in diet drinks and sugar-free products, may act as triggers for some.

Beyond "Don't Eat": Creative Substitutions:

The **Migraine Relief Plan and Cookbook** doesn't just tell you what to avoid; it empowers you with a delicious world of alternatives:

- Craving pizza? Swap processed dough for a whole-wheat cauliflower crust, top it with grilled chicken and colorful vegetables.
- Need a sweet treat? Indulge in a smoothie made with berries, spinach, and almond milk for a satisfying and nutritious burst.
- Yearning for comfort food? Whip up a lentil soup packed with protein and fiber, seasoned with fragrant herbs.

Remember, personalization is key. Consult your doctor or a registered dietitian to create a plan tailored to your unique needs and triggers. Keep a food diary to track your responses and discover your own personal migraine landscape.

Embrace the journey, explore the delicious possibilities, and empower yourself with knowledge. With your **Migraine Relief Plan and Cookbook** as your guide, you can navigate the food landscape, transform your relationship with food, and unlock a path towards a healthier, migraine-free future.

CHAPTER 3

Core Benefits of Following a Migraine Relief Plan and Cookbook:

1. Reduced Migraine Frequency and Intensity:

- **Identifying and avoiding triggers:** By pinpointing and minimizing trigger foods through this plan, you can significantly reduce the number of migraine attacks you experience.
- **Anti-inflammatory diet:** The emphasis on fruits, vegetables, whole grains, and lean protein reduces inflammation in the body, which can contribute to migraines.
- **Balanced nutrition:** Regular, balanced meals with sustained energy release help prevent blood sugar fluctuations, another potential trigger.

2. Improved Overall Health and Well-being:

- **Enhanced dietary choices:** Focusing on nutrient-rich foods promotes overall health, boosting your immune system, energy levels, and mood.
- **Reduced risk of chronic diseases:** The anti-inflammatory diet aligns with principles linked to

preventing heart disease, diabetes, and certain
cancers.

- **Healthy weight management:** Balanced meals and
portion control support healthy weight, which can
have a positive impact on migraine frequency in
some individuals.

3. Increased Quality of Life:

- **Reduced pain and discomfort:** Fewer migraines
translate to less pain, allowing you to engage in
activities you enjoy without fear of an attack.
- **Improved mood and cognitive function:** Chronic
pain can take a toll on mental well-being. Managing
migraines can elevate mood and sharpen cognitive
function.
- **Greater control and empowerment:**
Understanding your triggers and taking control of
your diet fosters a sense of empowerment and
improves self-confidence.

4. Delicious and Sustainable Approach:

- **Variety and flavor:** The cookbook offers an array
of delicious recipes catering to diverse preferences,
ensuring you don't feel deprived or limited.
- **Emphasis on whole foods:** The focus on real,
unprocessed ingredients encourages healthier and
more sustainable eating habits.

- **Meal plans and guidance:** The provided plans and expert tips make adapting to this approach easier and more manageable.

5. Tailored to Individual Needs:

- **Personalization:** The plan encourages identifying your unique triggers and incorporating them into your dietary choices.
- **Dietary support:** Consulting with a registered dietitian can ensure the plan aligns with your specific needs and health conditions.
- **Holistic approach:** The guide encourages combining dietary changes with stress management and other healthy habits for optimal results.

By embracing these core benefits, following a Migraine Relief Plan and Cookbook can become a transformative journey towards a healthier, happier, and migraine-free future. Remember, consistency and individual customization are key to unlocking the full potential of this approach.

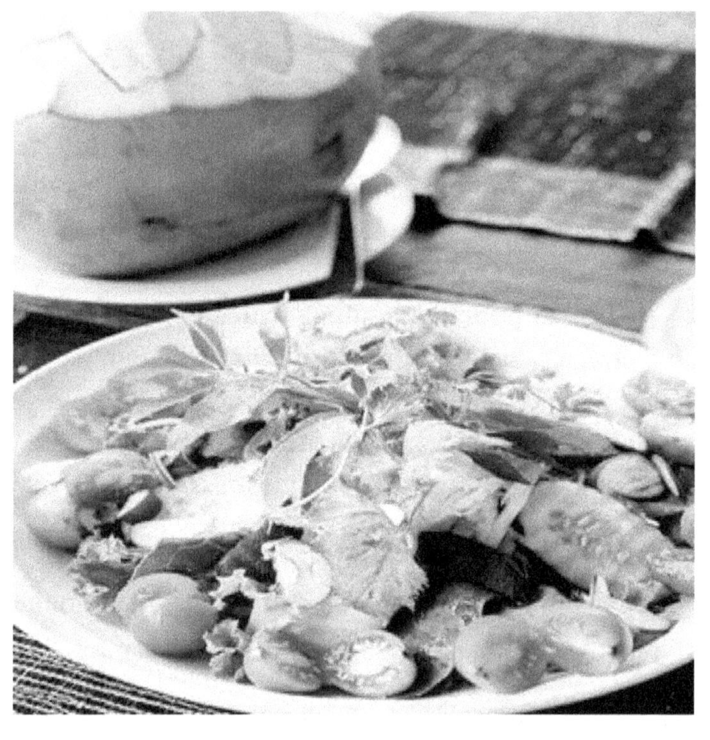

CHAPTER 4

Following Your Migraine Relief Plan and Cookbook: A Step-by-Step Guide

Embarking on a migraine-free journey with your Migraine Relief Plan and Cookbook requires commitment and understanding. Here's a step-by-step guide to get you started:

1. Understand the Science:

- **Read the introductory sections:** Familiarize yourself with the science behind migraines, the role of food as a trigger, and the benefits of the anti-inflammatory approach.
- **Discover your triggers:** Learn about common triggers and keep a food diary to identify any personal triggers you may have.

2. Embrace the Anti-Inflammatory Diet:

- **Prioritize fruits and vegetables:** Aim for 5-7 servings daily, choosing colors for a variety of nutrients.

- **Whole grains are your friends:** Incorporate brown rice, quinoa, oats, and whole-wheat bread for sustained energy and fiber.
- **Lean protein is key:** Chicken, fish, beans, and tofu provide essential nutrients without inflammatory effects.
- **Healthy fats matter:** Include avocados, nuts, seeds, and olive oil for brain health and inflammation reduction.
- **Explore spices and herbs:** Leverage turmeric, ginger, garlic, and rosemary for added flavor and anti-inflammatory benefits.

3. Minimize Potential Triggers:

- **Limit processed meats:** Minimize hot dogs, sausages, and deli meats due to potential nitrate and nitrite content.
- **Watch out for refined carbohydrates:** Reduce white bread, sugary cereals, and pastries to control blood sugar spikes.
- **Be cautious with aged cheeses:** Cheddar, blue cheese, and Parmesan contain tyramine, a potential trigger for some individuals.
- **Read labels for MSG:** Avoid monosodium glutamate often found in processed foods and Chinese cuisine if it's a trigger for you.
- **Consider artificial sweeteners:** If sensitive, opt for natural sweeteners or avoid them altogether.

4. Utilize the Cookbook:

- **Explore the recipes:** Discover delicious dishes aligned with the anti-inflammatory approach, catering to various dietary preferences.
- **Start with simple swaps:** Gradually replace trigger foods with healthier alternatives suggested in the recipes.
- **Plan your meals:** Utilize the weekly plans provided or create your own based on your needs and preferences.
- **Don't be afraid to adapt:** Substitute ingredients based on allergies or preferences, remembering the core principles.

5. Personalize and Seek Support:

- **Consult a healthcare professional:** Discuss your migraines, triggers, and the plan with your doctor or a registered dietitian for personalized guidance.
- **Join online communities:** Connect with others managing migraines for support, encouragement, and recipe inspiration.
- **Be patient and consistent:** Remember, results may take time. Celebrate small victories and don't get discouraged by setbacks.

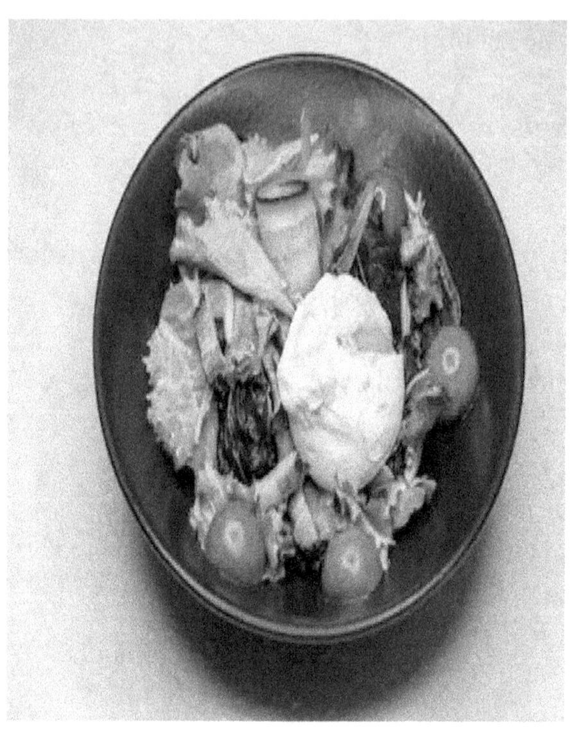

CHAPTER 5

20 Healthy Shopping Ingredients for Your Migraine Relief Plan and Cookbook:

Fruits and Vegetables:

1. **Leafy greens:** Spinach, kale, romaine lettuce (rich in magnesium and nitrates, potentially beneficial for migraines)
2. **Berries:** Blueberries, strawberries, raspberries (high in antioxidants with anti-inflammatory properties)
3. **Citrus fruits:** Oranges, grapefruits, lemons (packed with vitamin C and beneficial flavonoids)
4. **Avocados:** Healthy fats and antioxidants can support brain health and reduce inflammation.
5. **Bell peppers:** Various colors offer a range of vitamins and antioxidants.
6. **Broccoli:** Cruciferous vegetable with potential anti-inflammatory benefits.
7. **Sweet potatoes:** Rich in fiber and vitamin A, offering sustained energy.

Protein Sources:

8. **Fatty fish:** Salmon, tuna, mackerel (rich in omega-3 fatty acids with anti-inflammatory effects).
9. **Skinless chicken breasts:** Lean protein without inflammatory saturated fats.
10. **Lentils and beans:** Excellent source of plant-based protein and fiber.
11. **Eggs:** Good source of protein, choline, and vitamin D, important for brain health.
12. **Tofu and tempeh:** Versatile plant-based protein options for vegetarians and vegans.

Healthy Fats and Grains:

13. **Nuts and seeds:** Almonds, walnuts, chia seeds, flaxseeds (provide healthy fats, fiber, and omega-3s).
14. **Olive oil:** Extra virgin olive oil is a healthy source of monounsaturated fats.
15. **Quinoa:** A complete protein and gluten-free grain rich in antioxidants.
16. **Brown rice:** Whole-grain option with more fiber and nutrients than white rice.

Spices and Herbs:

17. **Ginger:** Known for its anti-inflammatory and nausea-reducing properties.

18. **Turmeric:** Curcumin, the active ingredient in turmeric, has anti-inflammatory effects.
19. **Garlic:** Potential benefits for reducing inflammation and blood pressure.
20. **Rosemary:** Antioxidant and anti-inflammatory properties, adding flavor to dishes.

CHAPTER 6

It's important to acknowledge that while following a migraine relief plan and cookbook like yours can offer significant benefits, there are potential complications if the right diet isn't adopted:

Nutritional Deficiencies:

- **Restrictive Approaches:** Focusing solely on eliminating trigger foods without proper guidance can lead to inadequate intake of essential nutrients, impacting overall health.
- **Imbalance of Macronutrients:** Not ensuring a balanced intake of protein, carbohydrates, and healthy fats can affect energy levels, satiety, and overall well-being.
- **Vitamin and Mineral Shortfalls:** Excluding certain food groups without proper substitutes could lead to deficiencies in vital vitamins and minerals.

Increased Frustration and Difficulty Adhering:

- **Strict and Unrealistic Expectations:** Setting unrealistic goals or expecting immediate results can lead to frustration and difficulty sticking to the plan.
- **Lack of Individualization:** A "one-size-fits-all" approach might not address individual triggers or preferences, making it harder to adapt and sustain.
- **Social Challenges:** Avoiding certain foods in social settings can be isolating and challenging, potentially leading to lapses and discouragement.

Potential Misdiagnoses and Self-Treatment:

- **Confusing Triggers:** Mistaking non-dietary factors for food triggers can lead to ineffective management and frustration.
- **Underlying Medical Conditions:** The plan might not be suitable for individuals with other medical conditions requiring specific dietary guidelines.
- **Delaying Proper Medical Attention:** Relying solely on dietary changes without seeking professional medical advice can delay diagnosis and treatment of other underlying causes.

It's crucial to approach your "Migraine Relief Plan and Cookbook" as a tool, not a miracle cure.

Here are some key points to remember:

- **Seek Professional Guidance:** Consult a registered dietitian or healthcare professional to personalize the plan based on your individual needs and triggers.
- **Gradual and Sustainable Changes:** Introduce dietary changes gradually and focus on building healthy habits for long-term success.
- **Balanced and Nutrient-Rich:** Ensure your diet includes a variety of whole foods from all food groups to prevent deficiencies.
- **Mindset and Support:** Prioritize a positive mindset and seek support from loved ones or online communities to stay motivated.
- **Remember, you're Not Alone:** Migraines are complex, and dietary changes might not be the only solution. Seek professional help for comprehensive management.

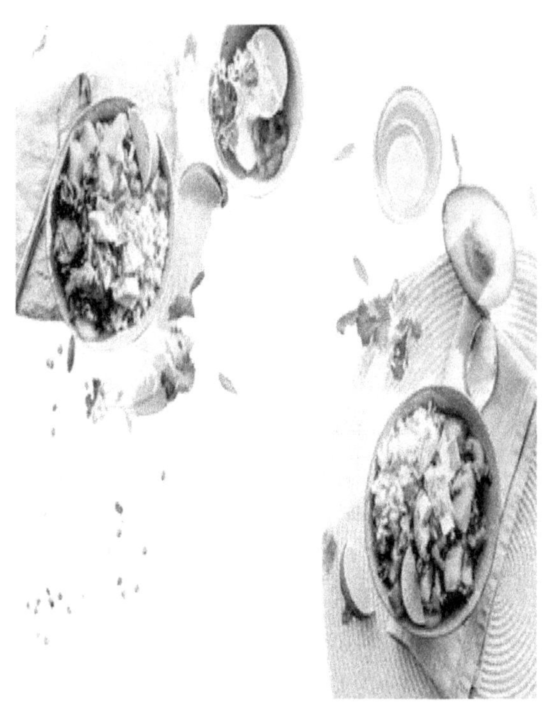

CHAPTER 7

Meal Planning for Your Migraine Relief Plan and Cookbook: A Recipe for Success

Planning your meals within the framework of your Migraine Relief Plan and Cookbook offers invaluable benefits for managing your migraines and overall well-being:

Reduced Triggers and Improved Control:

- **Proactive Approach:** Planning meals allows you to avoid potential trigger foods proactively, minimizing the risk of migraine attacks.
- **Balanced Nutrition:** Creating balanced meals ensures you're getting the essential nutrients your body needs for optimal health, which can contribute to fewer migraines.
- **Portion Control:** Meal planning helps manage portion sizes, preventing blood sugar spikes and crashes that can trigger migraines for some individuals.

Enhanced Convenience and Reduced Stress:

- **Decision Fatigue:** By having meals planned, you eliminate the daily "what to eat" dilemma, reducing stress and decision fatigue.
- **Time-Saving:** Planning helps utilize shopping time efficiently and streamline meal preparation, leaving you more time for relaxation.
- **Variety and Exploration:** Meal plans can encourage trying new recipes and incorporating diverse, anti-inflammatory ingredients into your diet.

Sustainable Healthy Habits and Empowerment:

- **Consistency is Key:** Planning fosters consistent adherence to the dietary guidelines, which is crucial for long-term benefits.
- **Sense of Control:** Taking charge of your meals empowers you to manage your migraines and improve your overall health.
- **Healthy Habits Spillover:** Meal planning can positively impact other aspects of your life, promoting healthy habits like grocery shopping and mindful eating.

Here are some tips for effective meal planning with your Migraine Relief Plan and Cookbook:

- **Utilize the provided weekly plans:** They offer a starting point and can be customized to your preferences and needs.
- **Integrate trigger tracking:** Mark trigger foods in the plans and actively avoid them when scheduling meals.
- **Consider different cooking methods:** Explore grilling, baking, and steaming for healthier options while enjoying variety.
- **Prepare ingredients in advance:** Chopping vegetables or marinating proteins beforehand saves time on busy days.
- **Involve family and friends:** Get them on board to create a supportive environment for your dietary changes.
- **Seek help if needed:** Consult a registered dietitian for personalized meal plans and guidance tailored to your specific triggers and health goals.

Remember, meal planning is a journey, not a destination. Experiment, adapt, and celebrate your progress. By embracing meal planning with your Migraine Relief Plan and Cookbook, you can empower yourself to take control of your migraines and unlock a future of improved health and well-being.

CHAPTER 8

14-Day Simple Migraine Relief Plan and Cookbook Meal Plan

Disclaimer: This is a sample meal plan and may not be suitable for everyone. Please consult with a healthcare professional or registered dietitian before making any major changes to your diet.

Remember: Adjust portion sizes and ingredients based on your individual needs and preferences. Identify and avoid your personal trigger foods while following this plan.

Key:

- **B:** Breakfast
- **L:** Lunch
- **D:** Dinner
- **S:** Snack

Day 1:

- **B:** Scrambled eggs with spinach and peppers, whole-wheat toast

- **L:** Leftover roasted chicken salad with mixed greens and avocado
- **D:** Salmon with roasted sweet potato and steamed broccoli
- **S:** Yogurt with berries and granola

Day 2:

- **B:** Smoothie with banana, spinach, almond milk, and protein powder
- **L:** Lentil soup with whole-wheat bread
- **D:** Turkey burger on a whole-wheat bun with sweet potato fries and side salad
- **S:** Apple slices with almond butter

Day 3:

- **B:** Oatmeal with chia seeds, berries, and nuts
- **L:** Tuna salad sandwich on whole-wheat bread with side salad
- **D:** Chicken stir-fry with brown rice and mixed vegetables
- **S:** Handful of almonds and grapes

Day 4:

- **B:** Whole-wheat pancakes with berries and maple syrup
- **L:** Leftover chicken stir-fry

- **D:** Baked tofu with roasted Brussels sprouts and quinoa
- **S:** Cottage cheese with sliced cucumber and tomatoes

Day 5:

- **B:** Greek yogurt with fruit and granola
- **L:** Black bean and corn salad with avocado and whole-wheat tortilla
- **D:** Salmon with roasted asparagus and quinoa
- **S:** Pear with string cheese

Day 6:

- **B:** Eggs Benedict with whole-wheat English muffin, spinach, and avocado (modify with smoked salmon or turkey if vegetarian)
- **L:** Leftover baked tofu with quinoa
- **D:** Chicken fajitas with whole-wheat tortillas, grilled peppers and onions, and black beans
- **S:** Carrot sticks with hummus

Day 7:

- **B:** Smoothie with mango, spinach, almond milk, and protein powder
- **L:** Chicken Caesar salad with whole-wheat croutons and light dressing
- **D:** Vegetarian chili with whole-wheat bread

- **S:** Apple slices with peanut butter

Day 8:

- **B:** Whole-wheat toast with avocado and scrambled eggs
- **L:** Tuna salad with mixed greens
- **D:** Shrimp scampi with whole-wheat pasta and steamed broccoli
- **S:** Handful of trail mix

Day 9:

- **B:** Quinoa porridge with berries and nuts
- **L:** Leftover vegetarian chili
- **D:** Turkey meatloaf with mashed sweet potatoes and steamed kale
- **S:** Yogurt with mixed nuts and seeds

Day 10:

- **B:** Protein pancakes with fruit and yogurt
- **L:** Salad with grilled chicken, avocado, and balsamic vinaigrette
- **D:** Salmon with roasted vegetables and brown rice
- **S:** Pear slices with almond butter

Day 11:

- **B:** Omelets with spinach, peppers, and cheese

- **L:** Lentil soup with whole-wheat bread
- **D:** Chicken stir-fry with brown rice and mixed vegetables
- **S:** Cottage cheese with pineapple chunks

Day 12:

- **B:** Smoothie with banana, spinach, almond milk, and protein powder
- **L:** Quinoa salad with black beans, corn, and avocado
- **D:** Baked tofu with roasted Brussels sprouts and quinoa
- **S:** Sliced cucumber with hummus

Day 13:

- **B:** Avocado toast with scrambled eggs
- **L:** Leftover chicken stir-fry
- **D:** Vegetarian chili with whole-wheat bread
- **S:** Apple slices with peanut butter

Day 14:

- **B:** Oatmeal with berries and nuts
- **L:** Chicken Caesar salad with whole-wheat croutons and light dressing
- **D:** Shrimp scampi with whole-wheat pasta and steamed broccoli
- **S:** Yogurt with mixed nuts and seeds

CONCLUSION

Embracing Empowerment: Your Journey to a Migraine-Free Future Begins Here

This is not just a cookbook; it's a transformative guide, an empowering key unlocking a door to a world where vibrant flavors dance with migraine relief. You've embarked on a journey of self-discovery, exploring the complex connection between food and migraines. Remember, this path is uniquely yours. Embrace the delicious possibilities, celebrate small victories, and never lose sight of your ultimate goal: a life unburdened by head pain.

The journey might not be linear. There will be days when cravings beckon, or social gatherings pose challenges. But with each step, you build resilience, refine your understanding of your triggers, and strengthen your commitment to well-being. Remember, consistency is key, but progress, not perfection, defines success. Adapt the recipes, explore substitutes, and personalize your approach.

Every healthy meal you prepare, every trigger you avoid, is a triumph, a brick laid on the foundation of your migraine-free future.

Think beyond just managing pain. Imagine the possibilities: waking up with clear skies in your head, embracing social events without fear, experiencing the full vibrancy of life, unhindered. Picture yourself thriving, not just surviving. This transformative journey opens doors to not just fewer migraines, but also improved energy, enhanced mood, and a deeper connection to your well-being.

Remember, you are not alone. This guide is your companion, but the power lies within you. Embrace the knowledge, experiment with the recipes, and personalize your approach. Trust the science, celebrate your progress, and never lose sight of the incredible future that awaits. With each delicious bite, you're not just nourishing your body, you're empowering yourself, reclaiming control, and writing a new chapter in your life: a migraine-free masterpiece. So, embark on this culinary adventure with confidence, knowing that every step brings you closer to a brighter, healthier, and ultimately, migraine-free you.